Secret Back Pain Cure

Cheryl Alker

WWW.SECRETBACKPAINCURE.COM
WWW.24SEVENWELLNESS.COM

STRETCH YOURSELF FREE FROM BACK, NECK & SHOULDER PAIN

CONTENTS

> Flexibility is the important link from a sedentary life to an active life
>
> The Stretch Results program will re-balance your body bringing it into ideal postural alignment together with full range of mobility at the joint or joint complex
>
> Stretch Results is a total muscular re-education

If you are reading this then you are more than likely one of the billions of people worldwide who are suffering with back, neck and shoulder pain today. You have probably had to miss work at least once as a result of the pain and you are a regular visitor to the doctor, chiropractor or therapist. You are also contributing to the staggering amount of money ($50 billion in the US alone)that is spent each year on back pain – and that is just for the more easily identified costs. You are probably taking some form of pain relief and you know you should be exercising but the lack of mobility and pain make it almost impossible to take part in a regular program.

How about this statistic though?

Most cases of back pain are mechanical or non-organic, meaning they are not caused by conditions such as inflammatory arthritis, infection, fracture or cancer.

So what is the number one cause of so much pain?

SHORT, TIGHT MUSCLES – the majority of people's back problems are a direct result of poor postural alignment.

It is that simple—the fact is that when muscles become short and tight they draw bones closer together resulting in poor posture, poor functionality, poor joint mobility and range of motion, pain and discomfort. Tight muscles will literally hold your body in a restricted position. When a joint is immobile it loses most of of its natural lubrication (synovial fluid) that is produced as a result of movement.

Tight muscles = poor mobility = pain and discomfort.

Pain and discomfort = poor mobility = even tighter muscles.

It really is a vicious circle!

The **STRETCH RESULTS** program can help.

Stretch Results is a pure stretch program that focuses on lengthening and elongating the muscles that affect postural alignment returning you to a more neutral position therefore regaining functional flexibility and mobility. A body that is able to move as it was intended is a body free from pain.

Today's lifestyle, for the majority of us, means that we sit for hours each day, week after week, month after month and year after year. This position will eventually force the body out of alignment, leading to lower and upper back problems, lack of energy, a collapsed ribcage, loss of waistline, loss of abdominal support, the shoulders rolling forward and the head sitting in an incorrect position.

The first diagram is how we should look for correct postural alignment, however, too many of us fit into the other categories with bones being forced out of neutral. You don't have to have a degree in anatomy to see how the three figures to the right would have major issues in their spine.

PROPER ALIGNMENT

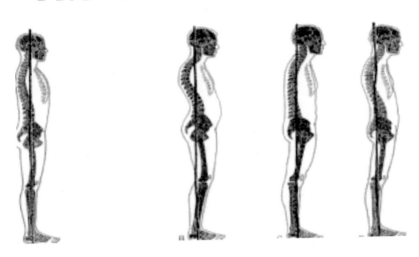

Let me give you an example of how when a muscle is short and tight it can cause back pain:-

We have a muscle called Iliopsoas. Iliopsoas is made up of psoas major and Iliacus and is one of our hip flexor muscles responsible for hip flexion i.e. lifting the leg to climb stairs. Sitting for long periods will shorten this muscle. Our muscles are attached to bone and originate in one area (the origin) and insert into another area (insertion). Psoas originates at the vertebrae in our lumbar region of our spine, it threads through our pelvis and attaches to our femur bone on the front of our leg. Now when this muscle is short and tight it will draw the pelvis into a posterior tilt i.e. your bottom will push back and the lower curve of your spine will deepen forcing your abdominals out. When your pelvis is being held in this restricted position day in day out the vertebrae in your lower back will be compressed causing the surrounding muscles to tighten causing pain and poor mobility in this area. Over time the gel within the discs will start to bulge causing herniation/slipped discs – now you really are in pain!

PSOAS
ILIACUS

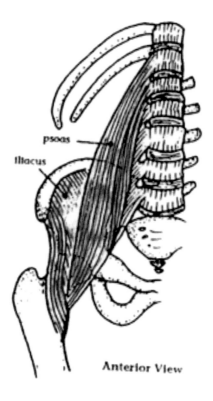

psoas

Iliacus

Anterior View

If you regularly stretch Psoas the muscle will allow the pelvis to sit in a more neutral position - you will regain mobility in the lower back, the gel within the discs will be massaged evenly around the disc avoiding bulging of the gel which may have been pressing on a nerve causing your pain and discomfort and your abdomen will pull in. A tight psoas goes hand in hand with weak abdominals and core support. Therefore improved flexibility will, not only result in reduced pain in the lumbar region of your spine but you will have a flatter abdomen!

On page 8 you will find a diagram with directions of the stretch you need to do on a daily basis if you believe Iliopsoas is tight.

[4]

Before you begin:-

- **Check with your Doctor or therapist.** Is it safe for you to stretch?
- **Warm up first.** Cold muscles will increase your risk of injury. Take a short brisk walk and mobilize your joints first or stretch after your work-out.
- **Hold stretches for at least one minute.** It takes time to lengthen tissues safely, also time must be allowed for correct alignment. Continually assess body alignment and learn to explore the muscle by changing leg arm or upper body position and weight applied.
- **Don't bounce.** Bouncing as you stretch can cause small tears in the muscle. These tears leave scar tissue as the muscle heals which tightens the muscle even further – making you less flexible and more prone to pain.
- **Focus on a pain-free stretch.** Expect to feel tension while you are stretching but not pain. You should take the stretch to the point where you feel tension and then hold it, the feeling should go away after approximately 20 seconds, however, if it increases and the leg starts to shake back off and start the process again but more slowly this time.
- **Relax and breathe freely.** Do not hold your breath while you are stretching results will be far greater if you increase the stretch towards the end of the out-breath. Ensure you breathe deeply focusing your breath towards the front, sides and back of your ribcage. This will encourage the diaphragm to work fully. Your diaphragm is your main breathing muscle and is attached to the lower ribs and lumbar region of your spine; it acts as a floor to your heart and lungs and a ceiling to your abdomen and internal organs. To access your breath utilizing the diaphragm fully you should inhale as fully as you can which will encourage the ribcage to lift and open whilst the diaphragm makes an opposite movement and starts to move downwards towards the abdominal cavity. When you exhale the diaphragm starts to lift and float upwards towards your sternum (breast bone) almost like an open parachute rising upward whilst your ribcage starts to close and moves downwards and inwards.

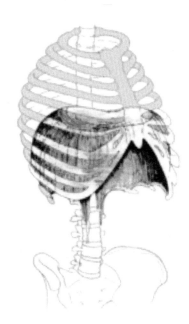

Before you try the stretch take this simple test:-

Lay on your back flat on the floor with both legs outstretched and your hands by your sides. Take a moment to analyze how your body feels in contact with the floor/mat i.e. if you were laying in warm sand what impression would your body leave? Analyze your head position, shoulders, upper and lower back, pelvis, backs of the legs, knees, calves and ankles. Analyze the two sides of the body does one side feel heavier, lighter, longer, or shorter? How do your legs fall, in or out? Does one side fall in a different position to the other? Pay particular attention to how much contact you have or don't have in the lumbar (lower) part of your spine. Once you have completed all the stretches return to this position and notice any differences with regard to the contact of your body to the floor.

Basic functional movement: Going up a step or walking up an incline.

The arrows on the stretches show you where you should drop weight and what parts of the body should be moving away from each other i.e. in the stretch for iliopsoas on the following page weight should be dropped through the pelvis but you should lift the upper body away from the outstretched leg.

BASIC LUNGE

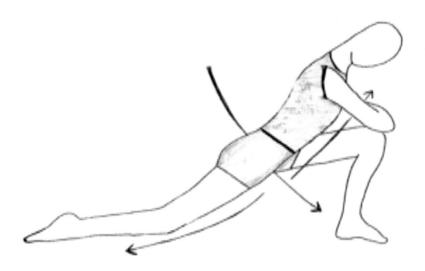

Position:

- Kneel on the floor. Bend the right leg creating a 90-degree angle in front of your body.
- Stabilize the foot flat on the floor.
- Ensure your right knee does not overshoot your toe.
- Extend your back leg fully.
- Stay upright with your chest lifted.
- Tilt your tailbone towards your navel. Rotate your back leg from your hip joint slightly inwards.

Note:

You may choose to use supports on either side i.e. yoga blocks, or a chair or bench placed in front of you. These you may also use to ease up the pressure on the pelvic area, by transferring some of your weight to your arm or arms.

If you find pressure on the knee of the extended leg uncomfortable place a cushion underneath for support.

Steps:

- Focus on the deep muscles of the hip area. To clarify this focus, place your left hand on the front of the hip of the extended leg, and the other on your right buttock (slightly above your tailbone).
- Breathe in.
- Move your hand on to the support. Create the stretch at the end of the out breath. Apply more body weight gradually through your pelvis to increase the stretch. You can press with the hand on your buttocks to help the forward movement of the tailbone towards your navel.
- Continue the stretch with the flow of your breath.
- For a deeper stretch hold onto a support i.e. chair, table, allowing further weight to drop onto the pelvis.
- Lift the head and drop the tailbone to the floor.

Hold the stretch for at least one minute, however, if you experience pain or it has been a long time since you stretched build the time you are in the stretch slowly.

Try to build the time spent in the stretch to two minutes.

Come out of the stretch gradually.

If you notice that your pelvis automatically drops to the side try and roll the pelvis into a more central position – remember the body will adopt a position that is familiar and comfortable – familiar and comfortable may be where it likes to be but where does it need to be for you to gain optimal results?

Remember to return to the floor after stretching both legs. Notice the difference of the contact in your lower back area, do you feel more contact? If you do you have just started your program to releasing this area from poor mobility and pain. Muscles have a memory, therefore if you continue to stretch daily your muscles will respond by remembering the new length and new position of the bones and short tight muscles, and continual pain will be a thing of the past!

If you do not experience a difference in contact, continue working with the stretch on a daily basis, the area may be particularly tight or your problems may be arising from a different muscle. Continual work with the program will highlight the areas that are tight by continual self-assessment before, during and after the stretches.

HALF MOON STRETCH

This stretch is for Quadratus Lumborum. As you can see from the diagram it is a very deep postural muscle that acts like two little pillars either side of the lumbar region of the spine and provides support. However, we know that when muscles are short and tight they draw bones closer together, therefore if this muscle is tight it will draw the ribcage closer to the pelvis resulting in a thicker waistline, a collapsed ribcage and referred pain to the lower back, hip and buttocks. One of its basic functional movements is bending sideways from sitting to pick up an object from the floor. Stretching this muscle will literally lift your posture and move your ribcage away from your pelvis resulting in a re-defined waistline creating space for the diaphragm to move through its' full range of movement and will assist with the release of compression through the lumbar region of your spine.

I strongly suggest you position yourself close to a mirror and then complete the stretch on the following page on one side. Once you have completed the stretch turn and face the mirror and look at the difference between the two shoulders. The results are often dramatic with a huge differential between the two sides, you almost feel as if you are going to topple over!

Basic functional movement: Bending sideways from sitting to pick up an object from the floor.

QUADRATUS LUMBORUM

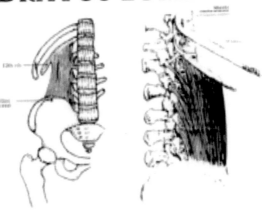

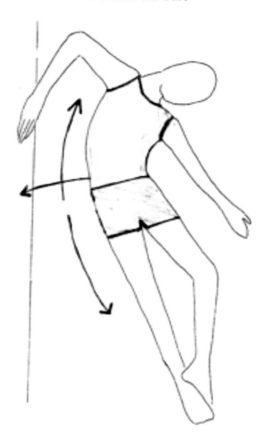

Position:

- Stand right side to a wall.
- Place the heel of your left foot over or on top of your right foot.
- Lift the right elbow upwards rotating it from the shoulder.
- Place the palm of your hand against the wall at a height which feels comfortable.
- Drop your head towards your left shoulder.
- Place your left hand on the right side of your lower ribcage.

Steps:

- Focus on your waistline and on increasing the space between your pelvis and ribcage.
- Create a deeper stretch by bending your supporting leg and arm.
- Breathe in to expand the side you are stretching.
- Create the stretch as you breathe out and the rise of the diaphragm lifts your ribs away from your pelvis.
- Further separate your ribs from your pelvis by dropping your weight towards your waistline. Be careful not to lean on your hand, your focus should be on pushing down into the heel of the hand.
- Continue the stretch with the flow of your breathing. Slowly extend your right leg, working against your anchor point. Keep your tailbone towards your navel.
- Once you have accessed your breathing towards the lowest part of the lung remove your hand and let the arm hang. Use the arm as an anchor point to assist in increasing the intensity of the stretch by easing it towards the floor.

As you become more proficient with this stretch, you will need less and less force in order to obtain an efficient stretch. Repeatedly define the concept of "waistline" to yourself. The target is to lift the lowest rib (and thus the ribcage) away from the pelvis. As you become more flexible in this area you will literally feel the movement of the bones sliding away from each other.

In order to reach the quadrates, the half-moon stretch requires a fairly diagonal positioning of the torso. Use the large back muscles, to gain access to the lateral sides of the abdominals when stretching. This is a very good stretch for people that are more mobile. Allow the stretch to travel into the quadriceps by bending and extending the legs.

Note:

Take a look in the mirror after completing this stretch. Notice your shoulder alignment – is one shoulder higher than the other? Check your waist, does one side look as if you have created more space between your pelvis and ribcage? You may now look lopsided but repeat the stretch on the other side and you will find you will match!

SEATED GLUTEAL STRETCH

This stretch targets the large gluteal muscle (the heaviest muscle in the body) together with the very much deeper Piriformis muscle. You will notice that the gluteal and piriformis attach to the sacrum. Now the sacroiliac joint moves and can often trap the sciatic nerve. This stretch is definitely for all you sufferers of sciatic pain, in fact, the pain you are experiencing is often referred to as Piriformis Syndrome.

Basic functional movement: Gluteus Maximus – Walking upstairs, rising from sitting

Piriformis – Taking first leg out of the car

PIRIFORMIS MUSCLE

Diagram indicates the proximity of the piriformis muscle to the sciatic nerve and how it can aggravate the nerve resulting in Piriformis Syndrome.

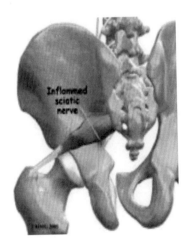

GLUTEUS MAXIMUS

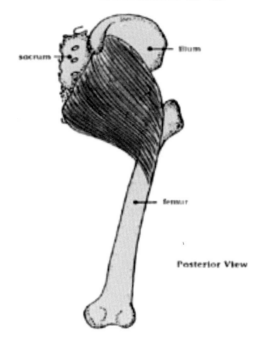

Posterior View

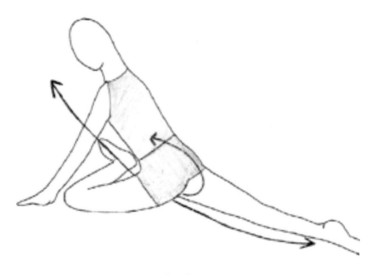

Position:

- Get into the basic lunge position, with the left leg bent in front, the other extended behind.
- Place your hands to the sides for support.
- Turn the knee of your front leg to the left on the floor.
- Move your foot to the right towards your centerline, and sit on your left buttock.
- Keep the back leg extended behind you, and turn it slightly in from the top of the leg.
- Move your pelvis into an upright position.
- Lean slightly forward, bending your arms.

Steps:

- Focus on the deeper buttock muscles, the sitting bone area, of the left side. Use your breath to open the lower back.
- Create the stretch while breathing out. Bend your arms to apply additional weight through the part of the buttock you are working on.
- Tilt the tailbone towards the ceiling to create distance between the bones.

Note:

Working from the inside out - in your mind travel from the inner thigh diagonally through the pelvis towards the buttocks. Imagine the buttock muscles sliding over the sitting bone toward the floor.

Variations

Keeping the pelvis where it is, move the upper body to the right and then the left to access different areas of the buttock and to follow the various direction of the muscle fibers.

If you have a knee joint problem you may find the standing gluteal stretch more comfortable.

[17]

STANDING GLUTEAL STRETCH

If the seated gluteal stretch is difficult for you to get into, then this stretch may be more suitable. The diagram shows the leg being lifted onto a barre; however, you can use the back/arm of a sofa or chair, a table, your bed in fact anywhere that you can comfortably raise your leg onto. You may find it more suitable to place a ball or cushion underneath the knee or shin area of the raised leg, particularly if you have poor mobility in the pelvis. Be aware that one side can be significantly tighter than the other.

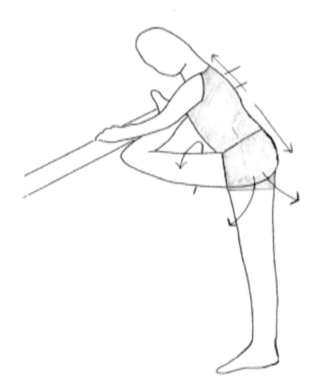

Position:

- Standing beside a barre, sofa, table etc., lift and bend your left leg up in front of you at waist height.
- Rest your foot and bent leg onto the surface and drop the knee to the left.
- Turn the standing leg in at the hip and keep your pelvis facing forward.
- Place your hands on the support, and tilt your tail bone away from your navel.
- Start to lower the upper body, keeping the chest lifted.
- Control your weight with your hands.

Steps:

- Focus on the deeper buttock muscles (the sitting bone area) of the left bent leg.
- Breathe in, and allow the lower back to expand.
- As you breathe out, engage your abdominal corset and tilt your tailbone further away from your navel i.e. away from you.
- Create the stretch with the opposition of movement. Bend your right, standing leg and turn your left knee further towards the floor. You will feel the stretch in your buttocks. Keep the sitting bones at the original height.
- Deepen the stretch by rotating your torso towards your leg that is on the barre and turn the supporting foot also towards the leg on the barre.

Note:

Take your time with this stretch. Since the muscles are deep and strong, it may take 10-20 seconds before you can even feel them.

Allow the weight to sit more on the foot of the standing leg.

Variations:

You can also use this stretch to mobilize your waistline and open up your lower back instead of the Half Moon Stretch. Lift the same arm as the bent leg and lift your lowest rib away for the hip, and tilt your ribcage further away from the bent leg instead of the buttocks. Focus on trying to create space between your lowest rib and hip bone in the lower back area.

If you have poor rotation place a ball or pillow underneath the knee of the bent leg to lift the leg a little you can use the ball as an anchor point.

Variation – If none of the above positions work for you this stretch still targets the muscles perfectly but it may be easier to achieve.

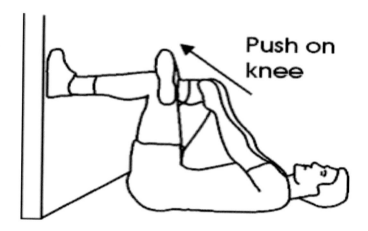

Steps

- Ensure your pelvis is in contact with the floor, so move away from the wall until this is achievable.
- Keep the ankle of the leg on the wall in line with your knee.
- The act of crossing the ankle over the knee may be enough stretch initially.
- Hold the position and then start to push the bent knee towards the wall until you feel the stretch and then hold.
- Ensure that the opposite side of the pelvis does not hitch up as you press on the knee, to create opposition you

need to maintain the pelvis to remain anchored and square.

- Use the breath and keep the upper body relaxed.
- Draw your navel towards your spine to provide internal stability.

LUNGE QUAD STRETCH – ANGLE 1

This stretch focuses on the large quad muscles, all variations should be completed as this targets the various insertion points of the four muscles that make up the quadriceps. If you find it difficult to balance please choose the position shown on page 27 with the supporting leg bent underneath you.

The quadriceps straightens the knee when rising from sitting, during walking and climbing.

Basic functional movement: Walking up stairs, cycling.

QUADRICEPS

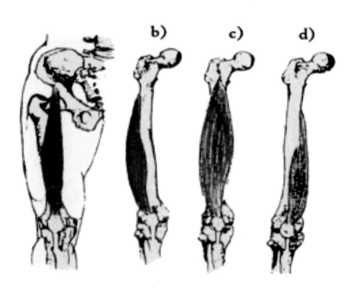

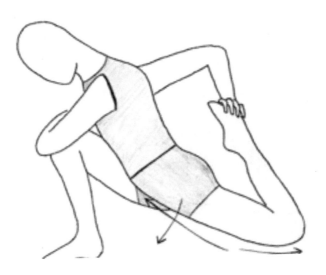

Position:

- Assume the Basic Lunge position.
- Use an appropriate support at chest height and something soft under the knee.
- Bring your right foot closer to your pelvis. Bend the knee of your left extended leg, and use the left arm to slowly pull the heel towards your buttock.
- Transfer your weight forward, away from your knee.
- Keep the left elbow up and fingers pointing down, grasping the toes.

Steps:

- Focus on the middle of your front thigh.

- Once you feel the muscle, lean further forward over the supporting foot. Create a deeper stretch by slowly bringing the foot of the left leg even closer to your buttocks. Keep tilting your tailbone towards your navel.
- Drop the weight onto the pelvis and let the supporting knee slide back.
- Lift the chest and head a little to further drop weight.

Note:

Be sure that you do not contract the hip flexor at the same time. The front thigh muscles have a strong biting point.

Contract your abdominals engaging the core so as to protect the lumbar region of the spine.

Ensure your front knee does not overshoot your toe.

Variations:

If you find it difficult to balance then bend the front leg underneath you (see diagram on page 27). Ensure no pressure is placed directly on the patella (knee cap) of the leg you are stretching. If you need to, place a cushion underneath the knee.

If you have difficulty reaching the foot, place a band around the ankle and ease the leg towards you by pulling gently on the band.

This stretch can also be done by lying on your side and pushing the foot into your hand and easing the pelvis forward or lying face down, holding the ankle and pushing the hip into the floor together with pushing the foot into your hand.

LUNGE QUAD STRETCH – ANGLE 2

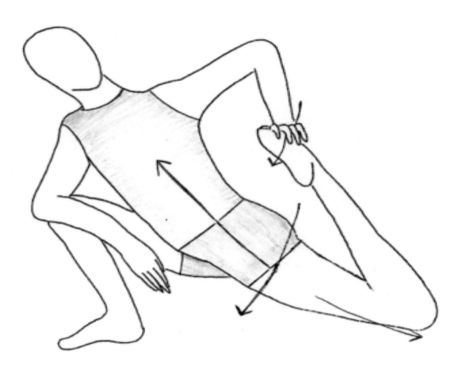

Position:

- Assume the Basic Lunge.
- Repeat as in angle 1, but keep the left elbow up and press the palm of the hand against the inside of the left foot.
- Keep foot alignment do not put undue stress onto the ligaments in the ankle.

Steps:

- Focus on the outside of the front of your thigh.
- Once you feel the muscle responding, lean further forward over the supporting foot. Create a deeper stretch by slowly pushing the foot of the left leg away to the side and then bring it slowly towards your buttocks. Keep tilting your tailbone towards your navel.
- Ensure the core is connected to protect the lumbar region of the spine.

LUNGE QUAD STRETCH – ANGLE 3

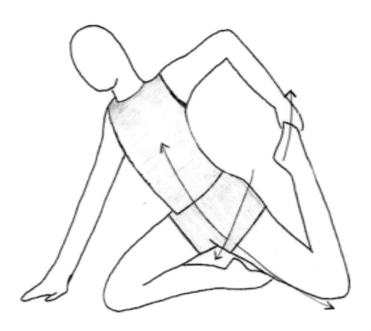

Position:

- Assume the Basic Lunge. Repeat as in Angle 1.
- This time press with your right hand towards the outside of your left foot.
- Bring your foot with your right hand towards the inside of your buttocks. At the same time turn your torso towards your right foot.

Steps:

- Focus on the inside of the front of your thigh.
- Once you feel the muscle responding, create a deeper stretch by slowly pulling the heel of the

Secret Back Pain Cure

right leg closer towards your buttocks, feeling the stretch inside the front thigh.

[28]

LAYING V

This stretch targets the adductor (inner thigh) muscles. The muscle originates from the front and back of the pelvis and brings the leg towards the centerline of the body, its basic functional movement is bringing the second leg in or out of the car. Its insertion point is all the way down the inside of the femur (leg) bone, from hip to knee, therefore you should not be too alarmed if you feel the pull around the knee joint.

Basic functional movement: Bringing second leg in or out of the car.

ADDUCTORS

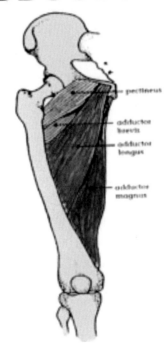

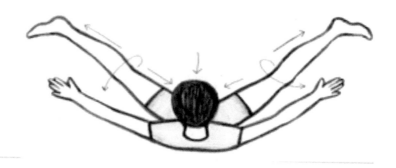

Position:

- Lie flat on your back with your head resting on the floor and your pelvis, legs and feet up against a wall.
- Open your legs to a "V" position.
- Keep the sitting bones at a 90-degree angle with the wall.
- Relax your weight on to the back of your pelvis.
- Ensure your pelvis remains in contact with the floor and the sitting bones in contact with the wall.

Steps:

- Focus on the inner thigh muscles.
- As you breathe out, lift your lower abdominal muscles but anchor your tailbone to the floor. Rotate the legs slightly further outward.
- Take a substantial amount of time with this stretch (2-5 minutes), and remember to relax.
- As you exhale soften your sternum/breastbone.

Note:

As your stretch continues, you may apply additional weight by placing your hands on the inner thighs and gently press downwards, according to what your range of rotation will allow.

If you feel the weight of the legs pull too heavily, place a ball or pillow under each leg.

To isolate each leg ease the left leg up to approximately 10 minutes to 12 and let the right leg drop. Repeat on the right leg bringing it to approximately 10 minutes past 12. Ensure that the opposing side of the pelvis does not pull off the floor, use your breath and try and anchor the pelvis down in opposition.

Bring the legs back to the starting "V" and notice if the legs have dropped a little further.

Remember if the legs start to shake or the burning sensation of the muscle intensifies the longer you hold the stretch, come out of it and maybe try again after a pause of 20 seconds or so.

Allow your arms to open out to the sides of the body in a "T" shape with palms up whilst you are relaxing in the stretch to encourage the shoulder girdle and chest to open.

When you have finished the stretch gently bring the legs together and bend the knees, placing a ball between the knees, give the ball a few squeezes, focus on the sacrum drawing inwards.

KNEELING HAMSTRING

For most people the hamstrings are without a doubt one of the tightest muscle groups in the body. Common problems that are caused as a result of tight/shortened hamstrings are low back pain, knee pain, leg length discrepancies and a restriction in walking/running. The pelvis will be dragged downwards to the knees and this can also cause roundness in the upper back causing discomfort in the upper back, neck and shoulder area. The drag on the upper back will force the head forward and could even be the cause of your TMJ dysfunction!

The diagram on page 33 shows one of the four variations you should do when stretching the hamstrings.

Basic functional movement: During running, the hamstrings slow down the leg at the end of its forward swing and prevent the trunk from flexing at the hip joint.

HAMSTRING

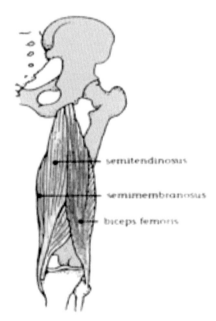

semitendinosus

semimembranosus

biceps femoris

[32]

Kneeling Hamstring (1)

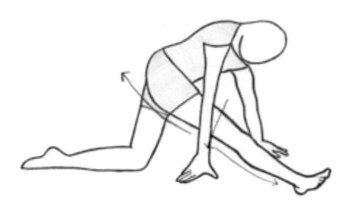

Start Position:

- Kneel on the mat, pelvis square.
- Extend one leg with the knee pointing toward the ceiling and the foot in neutral.
- Drop the weight through the pelvis so the sit bones are in line.
- Anchor your foot into the mat.
- Tilt your tailbone away from your heel.
- Lower your upper body weight and place both hands either side of the leg.

How to complete the Stretch:

- Gradually tilt your tailbone away from the heel as you use your heel as an anchor point.
- Continue to lower the body weight.
- Drop the weight through the pelvis.
- Press through the leg from the front of the thigh right through to the bulk of the

[33]

hamstring as if you were pushing from the inside out.

- Keep the pelvis square.
- Ensure the knee remains pointing towards the ceiling.

Note:

Remember the feeling/tightness of this stretch so you may compare to Kneeling Hamstring (2) and (3). If the pressure is too much on the supporting knee try placing a cushion underneath it or maybe the standing hamstring may be more suitable.

If the floor cannot be reached then use yoga blocks, a pile of books or small stools for support.

Engage your core to provide support for the lumbar region.

Kneeling Hamstring (2)

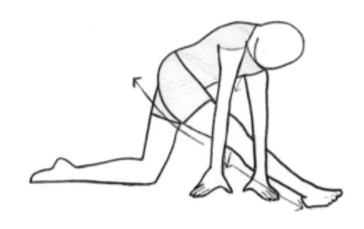

Start Position:

- Kneel on the mat, pelvis square.
- Extend one leg with the knee pointing toward the ceiling and the foot in neutral.
- Drop the weight through the pelvis so the sit bones are in line.
- Anchor your foot into the mat.
- Tilt your tailbone away from your heel.
- Lower your upper body weight and place both hands to the outside of the leg.
- Aim the upper body weight to the outside of the leg.
- This stretch can be a little uncomfortable and the leg will try to rotate outwards to stop the discomfort, do not allow the rotation, and keep the knee pointing to the ceiling.

How to complete the Stretch:

- Gradually tilt your tailbone away from the heel as you use your heel as an anchor point.
- Continue to lower the body weight.
- Drop the weight through the pelvis.
- Press through the leg from the front of the thigh right through to the bulk of the hamstring as if you were pushing from the inside out.
- Keep the pelvis square.
- Ensure the knee remains pointing towards the ceiling.

Note:

The insertion of this muscle can cause a nerve reaction and you may experience a tingling down the shin to the toes, if you do just point and flex the foot a few times and return to the stretch.

If the pressure is too much on the supporting knee try placing a cushion underneath it or maybe the standing hamstring may be more suitable.

If the floor cannot be reached then use yoga blocks, a pile of books or small stools for support.

Engage your core to provide support for the lumbar region.

Kneeling Hamstring (3)

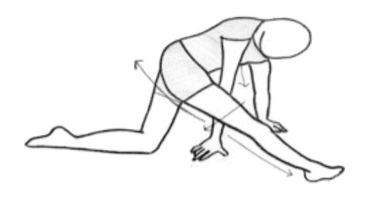

Start Position:

- Kneel on the mat, pelvis square.
- Extend one leg with the knee pointing toward the ceiling and the foot in neutral.
- Drop the weight through the pelvis so the sit bones are in line.
- Anchor your foot into the mat.
- Tilt your tailbone away from your heel.
- Lower your upper body weight and place both hands to the inside of the leg.
- Aim the upper body weight to the inside of the leg.

How to complete the Stretch:

- Gradually tilt your tailbone away from the heel as you use your heel as an anchor point.

[37]

- Continue to lower the body weight.
- Drop the weight through the pelvis.
- Press through the leg from the front of the thigh right through to the bulk of the hamstring as if you were pushing from the inside out.
- Keep the pelvis square.
- Ensure the knee remains pointing towards the ceiling.

Note:

If the pressure is too much on the supporting knee try placing a cushion underneath it or maybe the standing hamstring may be more suitable.

If the floor cannot be reached then use yoga blocks, a pile of books or small stools for support.

Engage your core to provide support for the lumbar region.

It is important that the above variations are completed so that you target each muscle within the group. If one muscle is shorter/tighter than the other three hip and knee joints can be affected.

The whole stretch should last approximately 2 minutes.

Variations:

If you are unable to touch the floor use yoga blocks or supports to place your hands.

If you experience pain on kneeling the laying hamstring stretch may be more suitable.

If you experience too much pain/discomfort in your lower back region, again the laying hamstring may be more suitable.

LAYING HAMSTRING

Before you do this stretch, lay on your back on the floor with both legs outstretched and hands by your side. Take a moment to close your eyes and notice the contact of the legs, pelvis and lower back on the mat. Once you have stretched one leg as below, lay it next to the other leg as before and feel the difference. Does your leg feel longer? Do you feel a difference in contact and weight? Does your body feel as if it is tilting? Does you pelvis feel lighter on that side? Check your head, has it drawn it into a more neutral position?

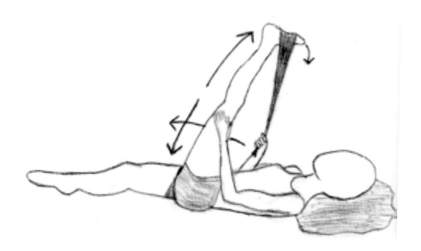

Position:

- Lay on your back.
- Either bend one knee or leave leg lying flat on the mat.

- Place a strong band around the other foot closer to the ball of the foot.
- If more comfortable place a cushion under your head.

Steps:

- Slowly lower the leg towards the floor and up again, no speed or momentum just testing range of motion, repeat 3 times.
- Hold the leg towards the ceiling and circle the leg several times to the right then left, keeping the leg passive in the band.
- Bring the leg back to center still with the heel facing the ceiling, hold the leg center and breathe in. As you exhale drop the weight onto your pelvis and feel the contact of the tailbone on the mat.
- At the end of exhalation, pause just before the in breath and push the heel towards the ceiling and toe towards your face, you will feel a "bite". Hold this position.
- Keep breathing and continuing to drop weight through the pelvis, focus on the leg lengthening. Do not push through the knee joint but focus on the bulk of the hamstring and calf and push from the front of the leg to the back.
- Repeat the circle again.
- Ease the leg across the midline of the body, towards the opposing shoulder; continue to drop weight through the pelvis.
- Bring back to center and continue with pushing through the heel.

If the other knee was bent when you started, lay this leg flat on the mat. Lower the leg in the band until it is approximately one inch off the mat circle a few times one way and then the other, turn the foot in and then out. Let the band go and lay the leg down next to the other one.

Analyze how this leg now feels, it may feel longer, lighter and you may be experiencing more contact with the floor.

BICEP EXTENSION

I am often asked for stretches that are good for neck and shoulder problems so the following are stretches that I have selected that are particularly targeted at this area. **Please be aware though, if your issues are in the neck and shoulder area, do not leave out the lower body stretches listed before.** Many shoulder girdle problems are as a direct result of the pelvis being out of alignment - the upper body has to adjust resulting in the pain and discomfort showing itself in this area but until the pelvis is neutrally aligned the upper body work will never be truly effective.

The first muscle we are stretching is the biceps which operates over three joints; it affects the shoulder blade, the shoulder joint and the elbow. It flexes the elbow joint as in picking up an object or bringing food to our mouth. It also supinates the forearm as in putting in the corkscrew and pulling out the cork. It also very weakly flexes the arm at the shoulder joint. When this muscle is chronically tight or shortened the elbow will not be able to fully be straightened and it will affect the position of the shoulder joint and blade.

There are two positions shown (Bicep Extension 1 and Bicep Extension 2) - you should do both.

Basic functional movement: Picking up an object. Bringing food to your mouth.

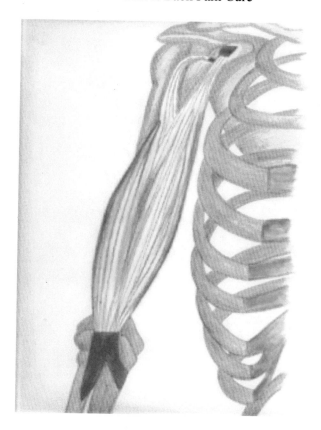

BICEP EXTENSION 1

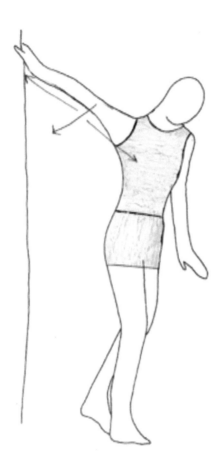

Position:

- Stand beside a wall; ensure you are close, approximately 1 to 2 inches away, but not leaning on the wall. Rotate your right arm backwards from the shoulder, dropping your elbow down.
- Place your palm against the wall at just above shoulder height.

[44]

- Lean on the thumb side of your palm. Step forward on the right leg, transferring weight onto it.
- Bend the knee and turn the foot inward.
- Be sure you maintain your alignment through the centerline.
- Allow your head to lower, and gradually, leading with the sternum/breast bone turn it to the left away from the arm.

Note:

Stay close to the wall but do not lean against it. This allows you to apply enough body weight through your arm while working on your stretch.

Keep your shoulder rotated upwards all through the stretch.

Steps:

- Focus on the bicep muscle, located at the front of your arm.
- Breathe in.
- While breathing out, create your stretch by rotating your torso away from your arm. Initiate the movement from your tailbone, and readjust your centerline.
- Turn your legs out, starting with the right foot, following with the left. Gradually bend your knees, working with your anchor point.
- Continue deepening the stretch, using the breathing, and further rotating the body and legs away from the arm.

Note:

Since this is a complex muscle in terms of ligament connections, you must use visualization to find the biceps. Once you can clearly feel the muscle, work slowly to deepen your stretch.

Once you have completely turned the body, take the stretch further by deepening the bend in your legs and gradually straighten the arm in this stretched position. Be sure not to lock the elbow, but work your way through the muscle.

Once you have completed the bicep stretch position 1 and 2 on one arm look in the mirror and see the difference between the shoulder and arm position of the stretched arm and the other arm. Is your stretched arm a little longer than the other one?

BICEP EXTENSION 2

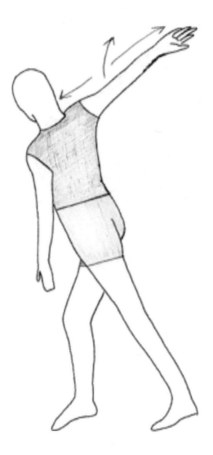

Position:

- Assume the same position as in Biceps Extension, but place the back of your hand against the wall.
- Work as Bicep Extension 1.

TRICEPS

The triceps originates from three heads and is the only muscle on the back of the arm. It extends (straightens) the arm at the elbow joint. Its basic functional movement is throwing objects or pushing a door shut and can be injured if you throw with excessive force. When this muscle is chronically tight the elbow cannot be fully flexed (bent). It will also affect the shoulder blade and its position.

Basic functional movement: Throwing object, pushing a door shut.

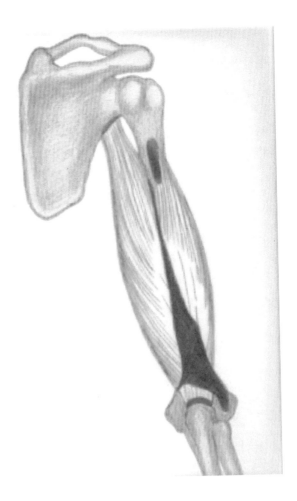

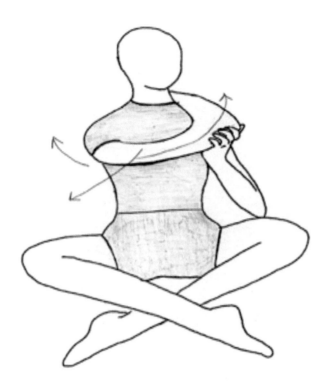

Position:

- Sit cross-legged on the floor in an upright position or in a chair with a straight back.
- Drop your weight on to your sitting bones.
- Bend the right arm, initiating the movement from the shoulder, and turn the elbow in.
- Keeping the arm passive, place the palm of the left hand underneath the elbow and then lift the arm across the body towards the left shoulder.
- Be sure the right arm remains passive.
- Relax the chest and drop your shoulders.

Variations:

[49]

Keeping your back upright is important. If sitting on a chair or against the wall, you can use a pillow against your lower back. If you find it difficult to locate an upright back position, do the stretch standing against the wall with feet parallel.

Steps:

- Focus on the triceps, located at the back of your arms.
- Breathe in.
- Create the stretch by gently pressing your right elbow to the left shoulder with your left hand. With the out breath, create opposition of movement by rotating your torso slightly to the right.
- Deepen the stretch by using your left hand to gently press the right arm closer to the body. Repeat breathing and rotation of the torso.

Note:

During the stretch keep checking that your right shoulder is down and the right arm is completely passive.

STANDING TRICEP EXTENSION

Position:

- Stand upright with parallel legs in a doorframe or next to a wall.
- Raise the right arm and rotate in from the elbow initiating the movement from your shoulder blade.
- Drop your hand behind your head, between your shoulder blades.
- Place the elbow against the wall.
- Allow the shoulder blade to drop further down against the back.
- Take your body weight off the left foot by crossing it in front of the right, bending the knee slightly.
- Gently rest the back of your head against the right arm behind you, keeping the length in your waist.
- Turn your head slightly to the left and focus your body weight into your right triceps.

Note:

During the stretch, anchor the shoulder blade down and relax your chest in order to isolate the triceps. Keep your feet close together.

Steps:

- Focus on the triceps.
- Breathe in.
- During the out breath, create the stretch by pulling your right elbow down towards your shoulder blade, keeping the right arm passive.
- Create the stretch by gradually bending the supporting right leg, carefully applying body weight to the triceps.

[51]

- As you bend your leg, create opposition of movement by rotating the ribcage away from the arm and inching the head a bit more to the left.
- Breathe out.

Note:

Continue with this process of breathing and creating opposition of movement. As the stretch deepens imagine the shoulder blade gradually moving down the back and separating from the arm which will lengthen the triceps.

Alternate your body weight between both legs to find the position most suitable for you to utilize your body weight.

STANDING TRICEP STRETCH VARIATION IMAGES

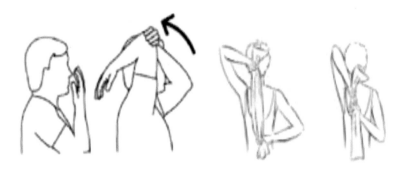

STANDING PECTORAL STRETCH

When Pectoral Major and minor are tight, the shoulders will roll forward, rounding the upper back, locking your trapezius muscle long and forcing the head too far forward. The result is neck and shoulder pain and possibly TMJ dysfunction (pain in the jaw). When this muscle is lengthened the chest and shoulder line will open, the breasts will be lifted and breathing capacity will improve increasing circulation to the head. This in turn will improve energy levels, neck and shoulder tension and headaches.

Basic functional movement: Clavicle portion –brings arm forwards and across the body as in applying deodorant to the opposite armpit.

Sternal portion: pulling something down from above, such as a rope in bell ringing.

PECTORALIS MAJOR

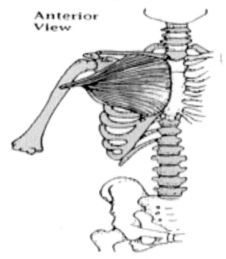

Anterior View

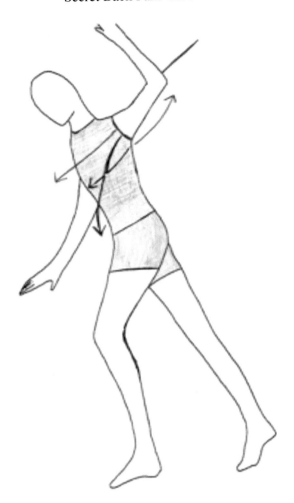

Position:

- Stand sideways in a doorframe or besides a wall half an arm's length away.
- Place your left forearm along the doorframe/ wall, elbow bent in line with your shoulder fingers up.
- Lean forward diagonally. Step forward with your left foot, and transfer your weight onto it.
- Bend your knee slightly. You can place your right hand on your chest to clarify the focus of the stretch.

Note:

The step forward creates opposition of movement for the stretch.

Steps:

- Focus on the chest and the shoulders.
- Breathe in.
- Create the stretch as you breathe out. Lean forward diagonally and take the muscle to its new length by further bending your legs.
- Now deepen the stretch by rotating your torso and head away from your left arm, initiating the movement from your sternum. Work with the stretch following the flow of your breath.

Now before stretching the other side, look in the mirror, notice the shoulder position compared with the other side. When this muscle is short and tight it will draw the shoulders forward, you will notice that one side is now higher or lower than the other side – this will depend on how far it has moved. Look at the distance you have now created between neck and the shoulder joint. You no longer see the roundness of the shoulder as it rolls forward - the shoulder line is more open.

KNEELING PECTORAL

This position will give a deeper stretch due to the use of body weight and gravity. I would advise beginning with the standing pectoral stretch and once increased flexibility has been gained in the chest area then you could try this more advanced position.

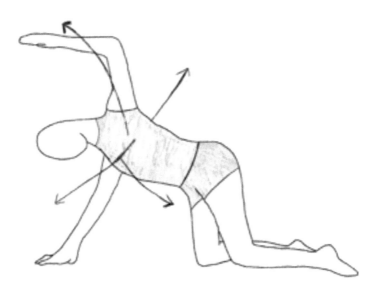

Position:

- Place your body next to a barre, wall, sofa or a table higher than torso level.
- Begin on your hands and knees, keeping your knees in line with your pelvis at a 90-degree angle.
- Lift the arm beside the sofa diagonally and place it on the sofa with the elbow bent.

Keep your weight on the supporting arm. Transfer the weight of your back forward.

[56]

Note:

Make sure your elbow is resting slightly higher than and ahead of your chest.

Steps:

- Focus on the chest.
- Breathe in.
- Create the stretch as you breathe out, and lean forward. By bending the supporting arm, you can gradually apply more body weight through the chest.
- Stay with the stretch and deepen it by concentrating on your breathing.
- Ensure your core is engaged so the lower back is not slumping.
- You can further deepen the stretch by turning the sternum away from your arm and then extending the inside leg back as you lean forward.

Note:

As you deepen the stretch, visualize the left shoulder blade moving back to aid in opening up the chest, and drop your head.

Variation:

For a more advanced stretch, focus on the deeper layer of chest muscles and extend the leg nearest the wall out behind you. You can alternate the positioning of your arm in order to isolate these muscles (for example, extending your arm forward).

If the kneeling position is uncomfortable on the knees then stretch the pectoral in the standing position as before.

LONG NECK STRETCH

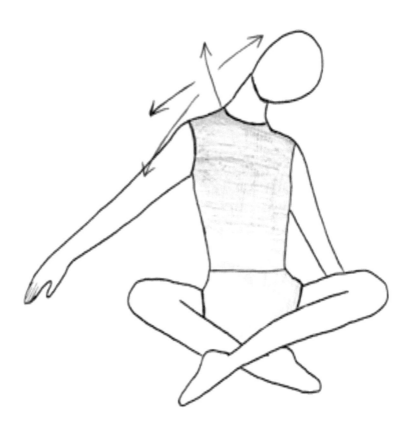

Position:

- Sit upright in a cross-legged position, or on a chair.
- Rotate your shoulders back and lift your chest upwards.
- Extend your left arm to the side, placing your hand on the floor.
- Tilt your head to the left, while lifting your cheek towards the ceiling.
- Relax your right arm.

Steps:

- Focus on the right side of the neck.
- Breathe in.
- Create the stretch and opposition of movement by reaching your right arm diagonally slightly behind your shoulder. Further relax your head to the left.
- Breathe out, emptying the upper part of your lungs. Keep your head in this relaxed position and deepen the stretch by slowly extending and lowering your right arm in slight movements.

Note:

Keep your weight even between both of the sitting bones. Allowing your head to lead the curve of the torso to the left will also add to the depth of your stretch. Continue rotating your shoulder back.

SIDE NECK STRETCH – FOR THE ANTERIOR AND SIDE NECK MUSCLES

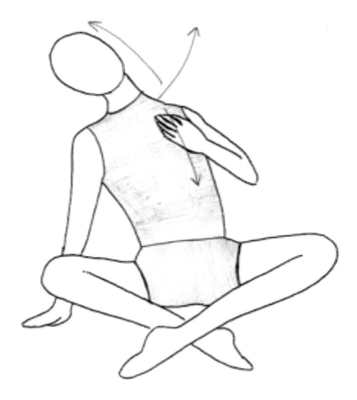

Position:

- Sit cross-legged on the floor with a straight back.
- Tilt your head to the left, lifting your cheek to the ceiling.
- Rotate your shoulders back and lift your chest upward.

- Place your left hand on your right collarbone and gently pull down the muscles around it.

Note:

Using your left hand to gently pull on the collarbone area helps to emphasize opening the right side of your neck.

Steps:

- Focus on the neck muscles running along the right side of your jaw line down to your collarbone.
- Breathe in.
- Create the stretch by relaxing your head and using your hands to gently pull and separate your head from your collarbone. Feel the opening of the side of your neck.
- As you breathe out, deepen the stretch further by lifting your right cheek further upwards.
- If you would like to progress the stretch, gently lower your left arm to the floor and behind your body. You may also use both hands on the muscles of the right collarbone area to deepen the stretch.
- Keep your weight even between both sitting bones.

CROSS-ARM NECK STRETCH

Position:

- Sit cross-legged on the floor or on a chair.
- Keep your back upright (see Note).
- Extend both arms down, palms up, rotate your elbows towards each other and cross right over the left.
- Lift your right arm with your left, underneath the elbow, keeping the elbows crossed. Place your left hand on your right wrist, palms facing each other.
- Tilt your head to the left.
- Be sure your right arm remains passive.
- Relax your ribcage and shoulders.

Variations:

The upright positioning of your back is important. If sitting on a chair or sitting against the wall, you can use a pillow against your lower back. If you find it difficult to locate a straight back position, do the stretch standing against the wall with feet parallel.

Steps:

- Focus on the muscles either at the side or back of your neck towards the shoulder blade area.
- Breathe in and focus your breath on your upper back.
- Breathe out and create the stretch by actively using your left hand to press your right arm down towards the floor. Relax your chest and drop your shoulders further down.
- Continue deepening the stretch by keeping your right arm passive as you slowly lift it up and down with the left arm. During the delay of your out

breath, gently press your right arm further down with your left hand.

CURVED NECK STRETCH

TRAPEZIUS

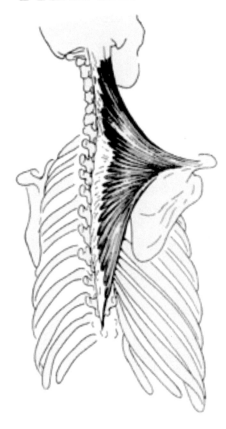

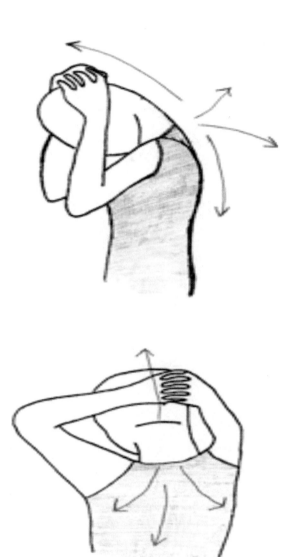

Position:

- Sit cross-legged and upright (See Note on positioning of Cross-Arm Neck Stretch), and focus forward.
- Create length in the back of your neck by tilting your chin down.
- Interlock your fingers and place both hands behind your head at a level above your ears.
- Bring your elbows together.
- Allow your neck, arms and upper back to be passive.

Steps:

- Focus on the back of your neck.
- Focus your breath between the shoulder blades.
- Create your stretch as you breathe out, using the weight of your arms to bring your chin closer to your chest. This will increase the curve of your upper back.
- Try to empty the upper part of your lungs, engaging your abdominal corset. This also creates opposition of movement. Allow the pressure of the next inhalation to deepen your stretch.
- Work on the stretch for a good length of time (a minimum of 3 minutes).

Note:

If this stretch feels as though it is creating too much pressure, you may ease it up at various intervals while you work towards a deeper stretch.

Vary the position of the head to the right and left diagonals.

PLATYSMA STRETCH

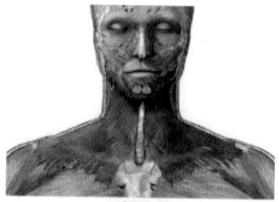

platysma

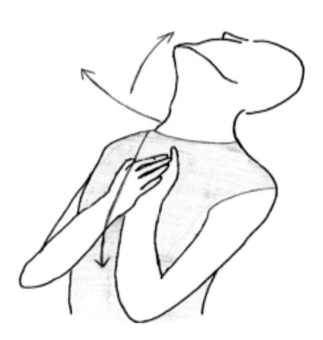

Position:

- Stand or sit cross-legged. Roll your shoulders back and drop them down.
- Lift your chest.
- Lengthen the front of your neck by slightly lifting your chin upward (do not close off the back of the neck).
- Place both your hands at the centre of your collarbone area, one on top of the other.

Steps:

- Focus on the neck muscles running from the top of your chest to your lower jaw line.
- Breathe in. As you breathe in, create the stretch and opposition of movement by using your hands at your collarbone area to pull your neck muscles down. To feel them sliding over your collarbone, further lift your chin.
- As you exhale, increase opposition of movement to deepen the stretch. To feel the stretch at the top of your throat, swallow.
- Continue focusing on the side of your jaw by turning your head slightly.

Note:

By swallowing you may become aware of the amount of tension you carry in the throat area underneath your chin. This stretch is suitable for addressing the tightness of the upper throat that results in a double chin. Do not pull the head too far back putting pressure in the cervical vertebrae; instead jut your jaw out more to increase the stretch.

PROGRAM

We are all aware that time is a precious commodity so over the next page we have detailed various programs you can follow depending on how much time you have on any given day.

Consistency is the key. Though your back pain is often the result of poor posture and poor movement quality, this has been developed over time and it will take time to re-educate good habits, it is absolutely achievable but I am afraid there are no shortcuts, repetition, repetition, and more repetition is the key.

If you believe you back pain started the instant you began to feel pain you are wrong, the pain you felt is the symptom, the cause, however, is most likely the result of wear and tear on your spine that has been exacerbated by long-term bad movement patterns that you now have to address, - it is time for a total muscular re-education and dealing with your flexibility issues is the first step.

Program 1

Ensure your muscles are warm and joints have been mobilized.

Choose the variation on each listed stretch that is suitable for you i.e. if the gluteal/piriformis stretch is better for you standing then this is the one you should use.

1. Laying Hamstring Stretch
2. Lunge Stretch – Iliopsoas – One Side Only
3. Seated Gluteal Stretch – Piriformis and Gluteal – One Side Only
4. Lunge Stretch – Iliopsoas – Other Side
5. Seated Gluteal Stretch – Other Side
6. Half Moon Stretch – Quadratus Lumborum – Right Side
7. Standing Pectorals Stretch – Pecs – Right Side
8. Half Moon Stretch – Quadratus Lumborum – Left Side
9. Standing Pectorals Stretch – Pecs – Left Side
10. Bicep Stretch – Right Side
11. Long Neck Stretch – Do This Stretch Standing – Right Side
12. Bicep Stretch – Left Side
13. Long Neck Stretch – Do This Stretch Standing – Left Side
14. Triceps Stretch – Right And Left

Program 2

[69]

1. Laying Hamstring Stretch
2. Quadriceps Stretch – One Side Only
3. Seated Gluteal Stretch – Piriformis and Gluteal – One Side Only
4. Quadriceps Stretch – Other Side
5. Seated Gluteal Stretch – Other Side
6. Laying V Stretch - Adductors
7. Half Moon Stretch –Quadratus Lumborum –Right Side
8. Standing Pectorals Stretch – Pecs – Right Side
9. Half Moon Stretch –Quadratus Lumborum – Left Side
10. Standing Pectorals Stretch – Pecs – Left Side
11. Bicep Stretch – Right Side
15. Bicep Stretch – Left Side
16. Platysma Stretch

Short Programs

1. Lunge Stretch – Iliopsoas – One Side
2. Kneeling Hamstring – One Side
3. Gluteal Stretch – One Side
4. Repeat All Three In This Order On The Other Side

1. Laying Hamstring – Both Legs
2. Laying V Stretch – Adductors
3. Laying Gluteal Stretch Against The Wall

4. Quadriceps Stretch – One Side
5. Gluteal Stretch – One Side
6. Hamstring Stretch – One Side
7. Repeat all of the above in order on the other side

1. Half Moon Stretch – Quadratus Lumborum – Right Side
2. Pectoral Stretch – Right Side
3. Half Moon Stretch – Quadratus Lumborum – Left Side
4. Pectoral Stretch - Left Side
5. Bicep Stretch - Right and Left Side

1. Pectorals Stretch – Both Sides
2. Bicep Stretch – Both Sides
3. Long Neck Stretch – Both Sides
4. Platysma Stretch

ABOUT THE AUTHOR

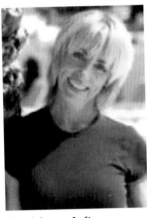

Secret Back Pain Cure was founded by Cheryl Alker as a result of her own lower/sciatic back pain issues.

Cheryl has worked in the health and wellbeing industry for the past 30 years. During that time she has helped world class athletes to people with hip replacements and everybody in between to achieve their specific goals. She also worked in corporate health, has lectured throughout Europe and the USA, is a health and fitness writer for many publications and has written training programs for the health and fitness industry that has been granted Continuing Education Credits with The Florida Board of Physical Therapy, the National Association of Sports Medicine, The American Council of Exercise and The National Association of Strength Training to name but a few. She has also worked with a United Kingdom Governmental backed program to train and certify exercise professionals. Working with so many people first hand gave her a huge insight into the staggering numbers of people suffering with back related issues but more importantly that back pain is indiscriminate, it can affect a world class athlete as much as it can an elderly sedentary person with a hip replacement.

Cheryl's back pain started during her first pregnancy and having been athletic all her life was shocked how debilitating the pain was but also how it affected her whole demeanor, being in constant pain caused severe depression.

Her wellness background allowed her to make educated decisions about how to relieve her sciatica and lower back pain but she soon became frustrated after finding that whilst she might get temporary relief from adjustments, medications, heat pads, massage, special pillows, the latest equipment she purchased, the pain always came back with a vengeance. Her bank balance was suffering as a result, and she was losing income with the time she was wasting making appointments and sitting in waiting rooms.

Relying on the "so called experts" a new product or cream on the market was not providing her with the answers she was looking for;

- "How can I relieve this pain?"
- "How can I manage?" it myself
- "How can I stop continually paying out thousands of dollars just to maintain the care

So she turned to her extensive anatomy and physiology background, the knowledge she had gained by training in so many aspects of health and fitness and the hundreds of people she had met along the way.

Secret Back Pain Cure was born - a truly holistic and natural approach that provides you with relief from any type of back, neck or shoulder pain. Cheryl wanted a program that would provide her with a proactive approach to managing her pain. The Secret Back Pain Cure package now provides you with the same freedom that she gained and she, along with literally thousands of others is living proof that this program could potentially change your life forever!

Made in the USA
Middletown, DE
19 September 2018